A Medical Guide to Hazardous Marine Life

A Medical Guide to Hazardous Marine Life

PAUL S. AUERBACH, M.D.

With Photos by

**The Author, Kenneth W. Kizer,
Larry Madin, and Carl Roessler
Front cover: Lion's mane jellyfish, photo by Larry Madin
Back cover: The author, photo by John Dunn**

SECOND EDITION

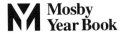 **Mosby
Year Book**

St. Louis   Baltimore   Boston   Chicago   London   Philadelphia   Sydney   Toronto

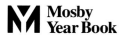
Mosby
Year Book
Dedicated to Publishing Excellence

Executive Editor: Richard A. Weimer
Developmental Editor: Rina A. Steinhauer
Project Supervisor: Jolynn Gower
Project Assistant: Pete Hausler
Book Design: Candace Fries, Gail Morey Hudson

Printed in the United States of America.

Mosby–Year Book, Inc.
11830 Westline Industrial Drive, St. Louis, MO 63146
GW/CD/WA 9 8 7 6 5 4 3 2 1

Library of Congress Cataloging in Publication Data
Auerbach, Paul S.
    A medical guide to hazardous marine life / Paul S. Auerbach ; with photos by the author, Kenneth W. Kizer, Larry Madin, and Carl Roessler. —2nd ed.
       p.   cm.
    Includes bibliographical references and index.
    ISBN 0-8016-6322-9
    1. Submarine medicine—Handbooks, manuals, etc.   2.   First aid in illness and injury—Handbooks, manuals, etc.   3.   Dangerous marine animals—Handbooks, manuals, etc.   4.   Marine toxins—Handbooks, manuals, etc.   I.   Title.
    [DNLM: 1.   First Aid—handbooks. 2.   Marine Biology—handbooks. 3.   Marine Toxins—poisoning—handbooks.   WD 401 A917m]
RC1005.A94   1991
616.02′52—dc20
DNLM/DLC
for Library of Congress
                                       91-15616
                                         CIP

FOREWORD

It is a privilege to introduce this guide book on hazardous marine life, in which Dr. Auerbach offers very practical advice for the special problems that scuba divers and other persons may experience in the unique setting of the marine environment. Although small in size, this book contains a large amount of important information for persons who may experience an unpleasant encounter with one of the denizens of the deep.

It has been my pleasure to travel with Dr. Auerbach to many exotic and remote corners of the world to teach groups of divers about hazardous marine life and other diving medical problems. In these wanderings, we have encountered a variety of medical problems that are rarely taught in medical school, first aid programs, or other similar training. For example, someone who has been seriously stung by a jellyfish while night diving in a distant corner of the Red Sea or who has suffered a deep coral cut on an out-of-the-way island in the Philippines presents special challenges for the best of physicians, let alone a diver having no special medical training. What Dr. Auerbach has done in these pages is to condense and organize a voluminous amount of information that would be helpful in situations like these and many others, and he has presented it in a way that it can be used by anyone. He has done an outstanding job in succinctly presenting therapies that may be lifesaving.

No guide book can ever be a substitute for professional medical training and experience, but that is just not always available when needed by those who venture under the sea. Thus, this book should be a very welcome guide to the diver, and should be stored in one's dive bag right next to the regulator and BC.

Kenneth W. Kizer, M.D., M.P.H.

Director, Department of Health Services
State of California
Sacramento, California

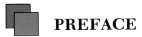

PREFACE

No matter how careful, every diver sooner or later is stung, bitten, or punctured by a hazardous marine animal. Carelessness and fatigue increase the likelihood of an unfortunate encounter. The cautious diver who is respectful of the environment generally can avoid major mishaps.

It is important for all aquatic enthusiasts to be knowledgable about appropriate first aid procedures that may be lifesaving if a victim suffers a major injury or adverse reaction to an envenomation. The undersea environment is unique in all aspects and so are some of the remedies described in this small book. The recommendations are current and conservative, offering the rescuer the best possible edge in caring for his companions and self. The guide is meant to be carried in a dive bag or first aid kit and is therefore not a lengthy discourse on the natural history, pathophysiology, and clinical pharmacology of hazardous marine animals. The references cited at the end of this book are listed for that information.

In all cases, seek professional medical attention when appropriate as soon as possible. The guide does not make you a doctor and should not substitute for definitive care in a facility that can provide advanced life support and a sterile environment.

Be safe and enjoy your diving. Remember that nearly all problems can be avoided by assuming a "look, but don't touch" attitude as you float and wonder at the marvelous scenery under the surface.

A Medical Guide to Hazardous Marine Life has proven to be a very valuable guidebook for divers, boaters, windsurfers, ocean bathers, and other marine aquatic enthusiasts. It has been gratifying to learn of persons who followed the advice written within its pages, and were able to successfully treat themselves or companions.

For the sake of the first-time reader, it is important to offer the reminder that the therapies recommended represent conservative methods ascribed to by most recognized authorities who manage marine bites and stings. Of course, there are occasionally local remedies that are also useful, but the reader can be comfortable that the advice offered in this book is safe and clinically proven, to the extent of what we know at the time of this writing.

In overall considerations of aquatic safety, one must be prepared to cope with near drowning, sun exposure, heat illness, hypothermia, scuba diving-related disorders (e.g., bends and air embolism), infectious diarrhea, motion sickness, and other problems that are beyond the scope of this particular book. A wise person carries adequate first aid supplies and acquires the necessary education before ever dipping a toe in the water.

My special thanks to Rick Weimer at Mosby–Year Book, Ken Kizer, Larry Madin, Carl Roessler, Chris Wacholz at the Divers Alert Network (DAN), and Rene Hugenschmidt of Hugyfot in Switzerland.

Paul S. Auerbach, M.D., M.S.

Associate Professor of Surgery and Medicine
Chief, Division of Emergency Medicine
Vanderbilt University Medical Center
Nashville, Tennessee

CONTENTS

A Medical Guide to
Hazardous Marine Life

GENERAL INFORMATION

CLEANING WOUNDS

Wounds that are acquired in the marine environment are often contaminated with seawater, sand, bacteria from the marine animal, venom, and other organic matter. To minimize the infection risk, they should all be cleaned as best as possible.

1. Control bleeding and attend to other life-threatening conditions (see Shark Attacks, p. 7).
2. Irrigate the wound with at least a liter (quart) of the cleanest disinfected fresh water available. If sterile saline solution or water is unavailable, use tap water or disinfected drinking water. There is no absolute need to add disinfectants to the water. The addition of povidone-iodine (Betadine) to the irrigation fluid is not harmful to the tissues if it does not exceed a 5% to 10% concentration, and it may help to kill bacteria. Never add solvents. Ocean water should be used only as a last resort because it is generally laden with marine bacteria. Remember, fire coral, anemone, hydroid, and jellyfish (coelenterate) stings should be detoxified with vinegar before the application of fresh water (see Jellyfish Stings, p. 27).
3. Remove all obvious fragments such as coral, seaweed, and fish spines.
4. Scrub the wound vigorously with soap and water. Do not pour alcohol, full strength antiseptics, or hydrogen peroxide directly into a wound. Remove any obvious debris. Rinse the wound thoroughly.

MARINE INFECTIONS

Wounds acquired in the marine environment frequently become infected. The bacteria that thrive in ocean water are often different from those found on land and can cause serious illnesses if allowed to proliferate in a wound. Therefore it is important to administer antibiotics early whenever there is a risk of infection. Apply these rules:

1. The best antibiotics to use are trimethoprim-sulfamethoxazole (Bactrim or Septra) in an adult dose of one double-strength tablet by mouth every 12 hours (or twice a day) *or* tetracycline in an adult dose of 500 mg by mouth every 6 hours (or four times a day). Another excellent antibiotic is ciprofloxacin (Cipro) in an adult dose of 500 mg by mouth every 12 hours (or two times a day). Any of these antibiotics might cause a "photosensitive" person to be more prone to a severe sunburn, so caution (and an adequate sunscreen with an SPF of 15 or greater) must be used during conditions of ultraviolet (sun) exposure. Always ask the victim whether he is allergic

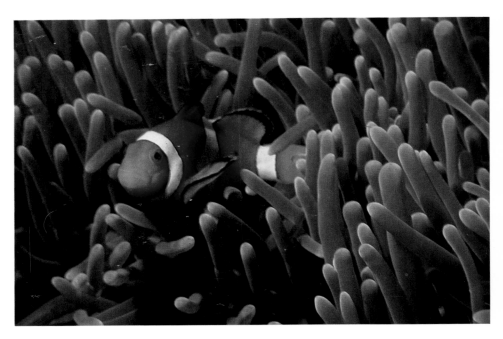

Clownfish with sea anemone (Kizer)

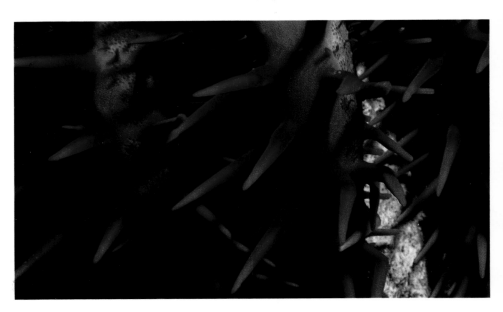

Crown-of-thorns starfish spines (Auerbach)

to any medications; if he specifies an allergy to "sulfa drugs," then tri-methoprim-sulfamethoxazole should not be used. If he is allergic to "quin-olones," then ciprofloxacin should not be used. *Any time a person has an allergic reaction (see below) to a medication, it should be discontinued immediately.* Popular antibiotics that are far less effective for many marine infections are penicillin, erythromycin, and cephalexin.

2. If a wound appears infected, administer antibiotics for 7 to 10 days or until the wound is healed. Signs of infection include redness, swelling, pain, a cream-yellow or green discharge (pus), foul odor, swollen lymph nodes (glands), red streaking in the skin from the wound in a direction toward the heart, and fever. Each day, scrub the infected wound vigorously with soap and water and apply a clean, dry bandage. Do not be concerned if the bandage sticks to the wound. A thin layer of antiseptic ointment, such as bacitracin, may be applied.

3. If a wound is new and minor (e.g., superficial coral cut, bristle worm sting, or swim fin blister) and the victim does not have an impaired immune system (i.e., is a normal host), antibiotics are not required until and unless an infection appears.

4. If a wound is new and major (e.g., a full-thickness [visible fat, muscle, or bone] cut, deep sea urchin puncture, stingray envenomation, shark or barracuda bite, or propeller injury) and physician medical care will be delayed for 48 hours or more, antibiotics should be administered for 7 to 10 days or until the wound is healed.

5. If the victim has an impaired immune system (e.g., diabetes, hemophilia, leukemia, acquired immunodeficiency syndrome (AIDS), or liver disease

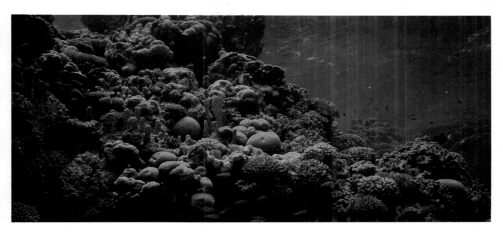

Coral scene (Auerbach)

or has undergone recent chemotherapy or long-term corticosteroid therapy), antibiotics should be administered as soon as possible following *any* wound (minor or major) and continued for 7 days or until the wound is healed.

6. To avoid infections, scrub all new wounds vigorously with soap and fresh water as soon as possible. Unless necessary for control of bleeding, do not cover wounds tightly with heavy layers of bandages. *Never sew (suture) wounds closed that have been acquired in the ocean or that have been contaminated with seawater* unless it is necessary to allow evacuation or to halt otherwise uncontrollable bleeding (is lifesaving). Tightly closing a wound that carries bacteria "seals them in" and increases the chance for an infection. If you must bring wound edges together, it is more safely accomplished with butterfly bandages or adhesive tape (e.g., Steri-Strips).

7. *Fish handler's disease:* When cleaning fish or shellfish, small nicks or scrapes are frequently acquired on the hands and fingers. If these become infected with the bacteria *Erysipelothrix rhusiopathiae*, a typical skin rash may develop within 2 to 7 days. It appears as a red- to violet-colored circular area of raised skin surrounding the puncture wound, with warmth, slight tenderness, and a sharply defined border. There may be an area of central clearing within the reddened perimeter. If fish handler's disease is suspected, erythromycin (333 mg by mouth three times a day), penicillin VK (250 mg by mouth four times a day), or cephalexin (Keflex) (250 mg by mouth four times a day) should be administered.

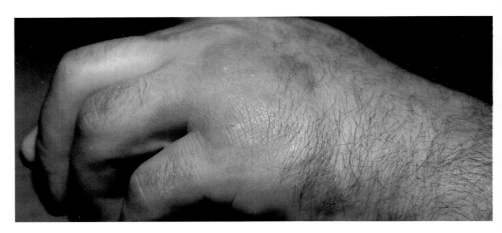

Fish handler's infection (Auerbach)

8. Make certain that your antitetanus (lockjaw) immunization is up to date before any dive trip.

ALLERGIC REACTION

Although most allergic reactions are minor, a severe episode can be life-threatening. Allergy follows exposure to animal venoms, plant products, medications, or any other substance to which the victim's immune system has been sensitized. Signs and symptoms of an allergic reaction include a low blood pressure level (shock); difficulty breathing (resembling asthma) with wheezing; swelling of the lips, tongue, throat, and vocal cords (which may obstruct the airway); itching; hives (red, raised skin welts that occur singly or in clusters); nausea and vomiting; abdominal pain; diarrhea; fatigue; seizures; and abnormal heart rhythms. The most common life-threatening problem is airway obstruction that accompanies facial swelling. *The rescuer should act swiftly at the earliest sign of allergic reaction*. Signs of allergic reaction include the following:

1. If the victim develops a swollen tongue or lips, hives, shortness of breath, profound weakness, or appears to be deteriorating, *immediately administer epinephrine* (adrenalin), which specifically counteracts the allergic reaction. Aqueous epinephrine 1:1000 should be injected just under the skin (subcutaneously) in a dose of 0.3 to 0.5 mL (milliliters) for adults and 0.01 mL/kg (kilogram or 2.2 pounds) for children up to the age of 12 years (not to exceed 0.3 mL). Epinephrine is available in allergy kits (Ana-Kit, made by Holister Stier, or EpiPen/Epipen Jr., made by Center Laboratories) with instructions for use. These require a prescription from a physician. *Anyone known to have severe allergies who travels outdoors away from medical care should carry injectable epinephrine*. Inhalable epinephrine mists available in over-the-counter products should not be relied on in a critical situation.
2. A drug that may be used for a milder reaction is diphenhydramine (Benadryl), which is administered by mouth. The adult dose is 25 to 50 mg every 4 to 6 hours; the child's dose is 1 mg/kg. Nonsedating alternatives are terfenadine (Seldane) (adult dose, 60 mg every 8 to 12 hours) or astemizole (Hismanal) (adult dose, 10 mg once a day).
3. Administer corticosteroids for a severe reaction. Prednisone tablets in a dose of 50 mg should be given to adults; the pediatric dose is 1 mg/kg. The onset of action of steroids is delayed for 4 to 6 hours. Repeat the dose the next morning if the victim remains uncomfortable and symptoms continue (hives, swelling, fever, fatigue, or diarrhea).

DIVER'S FIRST AID KIT

The first aid kit should be designed according to the number of members in the travel party, medical training of the party leaders, and distance from sophisticated medical care. Basic supplies that might be necessary to manage hazardous marine animal encounters include:

Medical guidebook
Elastic cloth bandages (Band-Aids), assorted sizes
Butterfly bandages or Steri-Strips, assorted sizes
2 × 2-inch sterile gauze pads
4 × 4-inch sterile gauze pads
8 × 12-inch sterile gauze pads
2-inch rolled gauze
4-inch rolled gauze
2-inch elastic wrap or conforming rolled bandage
4-inch elastic wrap or conforming rolled bandage
1-inch rolled adhesive tape
Scissors
Forceps (splinter)
Thermometer
Soap
Cotton swabs
1-ounce sterile eyewash
Tincture of benzoin (bandage adhesive)
Bacitracin ointment
Hydrocortisone cream, ointment, or lotion (0.5% to 1%)
Acetaminophen (325 mg) with codeine (30 mg) tablets (pain medicine)
Prednisone, 10 mg tablets
Tetracycline, 500 mg capsules
Trimethoprim-sulfamethoxazole (Bactrim or Septra) double-strength tablets
Ciprofloxacin (Cipro), 500 mg tablets
Erythromycin, 333 mg tablets, penicillin VK, 250 mg tablets, or cephalexin
  (Keflex), 250 mg tablets
Sunscreen (SPF 15 or greater)
Allergy kit: epinephrine with needle/syringe (Ana-Kit or EpiPen), diphen-
  hydramine (Benadryl), 25 mg capsules, or alternative such as terfenadine
  (Seldane)
Povidone-iodine 10% solution
Acetic acid 5% (vinegar)
Isopropyl alcohol 40% to 70%
Hydrogen peroxide
Instant heat pack
Snake bite suction device (The Extractor)

SHARK ATTACKS

1. Stay as calm as possible. The victim should exit the water as soon as possible.
2. Apply pressure *directly* over any areas that are bleeding. You can accomplish this by using a thick folded cloth under the palm or heel of your hand, a stack of gauze squares under an elastic wrap, or your bare fingers. If the bandage soaks through, unwrap it and make certain that it is positioned directly over the bleeding site. Almost all bleeding stops with direct pressure. After you begin to apply pressure, don't peek underneath (thus releasing pressure) for at least 10 minutes to give the blood a chance to begin to clot, blood vessels to contract, and the bleeding to cease. Applying a cold pack over the compress may hasten the process. Scalp wounds tend to bleed freely and may require prolonged pressure.
3. Have the victim lie down and elevate the injured part above the level of the heart.
4. If you apply a pressure dressing with bandages or cloth, do not apply the dressing so tightly that circulation beyond the dressing is affected. Make certain that the fingertips and toes remain pink (not blue) and that the digits do not go numb.
5. Prolonged uncontrollable bleeding is rare unless an amputation has occurred or a major blood vessel is torn. Applying extreme compression to "pressure points"—radial (wrist), brachial (elbow), femoral (groin) arteries—stops nearly *all* circulation beyond the pressure, so it is effectively the same as applying a tourniquet. *Tourniquets are extremely hazardous and indicated only in life-threatening situations when properly applied by experienced persons*. The decision to apply a tourniquet is one in which a limb may be sacrificed to save the victim's life. The tourniquet is applied to the limb between the bleeding site and the heart, as close to the injury as possible, and tightened just to the point at which bleeding can be controlled with direct pressure over the wound. *The tourniquet should be released briefly every 10 to 15 minutes to see if it is still necessary*.
6. If the bleeding is from a severe cut in the neck, do not disturb the wound, because disrupting a blood clot may initiate severe bleeding. Apply a firm pressure dressing (without choking the victim).
7. If there is a cut through which internal organs or bones are protruding, do not attempt to push these back inside. Cover them with continually moistened bandages held in place without excess pressure.

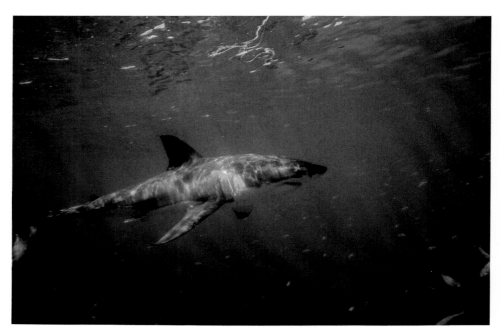

Great white shark (Roessler)

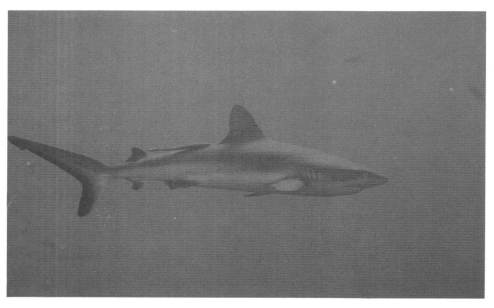

Reef shark (Auerbach)

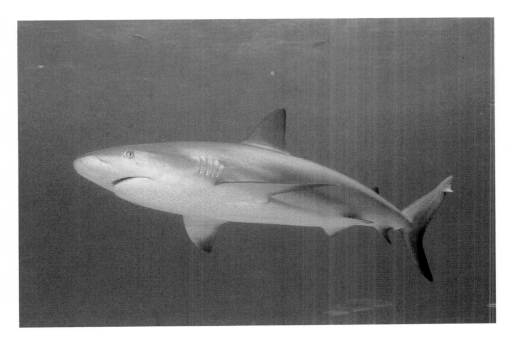

Black-tipped reef shark (Dean McInnis)

8. If the chest cavity is entered, all open wounds should be rapidly covered, particularly if they are "bubbling."
9. After you have controlled the bleeding, keep the injured part from moving. This may be accomplished with preformed or improvised splints. Be certain to pad all body parts within the splints. Check all dressings regularly to be certain that swelling underneath has not made them too tight.
10. If the victim's skin is abraded from a shark "bumping," control bleeding, scrub with soap and water, then rinse the skin well with clean fresh water (use ocean water only as a last resort). Apply an antiseptic ointment (such as bacitracin) and cover loosely with a sterile dressing.
11. If the wound shows signs of infection, administer antibiotics (see Marine Infections, p. 1).

SHARK AVOIDANCE AND REPULSION

There are times when a diver doesn't wish to encounter sharks, particularly those notorious for aggressive behavior towards humans. Generally accepted recommendations for shark avoidance and repulsion include the following:

1. Shark-infested water should be avoided, particularly at dusk and in the early evening. Avoid water that has been posted as containing hazardous sharks. Do not swim with animals, such as dogs and horses, in shark-infested water. Do not remain in the water with sharks if you are overly fearful.
2. Swimmers and divers should remain in groups, as sharks tend to attack isolated individuals. Be vigilant for the presence of sharks.
3. Avoid swimming or diving in turbid water, drop-offs, deep channels, and near sanitation waste outlets, as these are areas often frequented by larger sharks.
4. Do not bleed freely into the water in the vicinity of hazardous sharks. If you sustain a cut in the water, wrap it if possible and leave the water.
5. Captured fish must be removed from the water as soon as possible or tethered at a considerable distance from any divers or spear fishermen. There is no greater attractant for a shark than fish blood.
6. Do not wear shiny gear that will simulate a fishing lure.
7. The presence of porpoises or sea lions in the water does not preclude the presence of sharks. Be alert for the presence of a shark whenever schools of fish behave in an erratic manner.
8. Do not tease or corner a shark. If a shark begins to act in an agitated manner, do not photograph it at close range using a strobe flash apparatus. Leave shark feeding to experts.
9. If a shark appears in shallow water, leave the area with slow, purposeful movements, facing the shark if possible and avoiding panicked behavior. If a shark approaches in deep water, the diver should remain submerged. Do not surface rapidly. *Do not splash the water's surface or create any underwater commotion that might cause a shark to interpret your behavior as that of a struggling fish*. Move to defensive terrain with posterior protection (e.g., snuggle up to a coral head or wall) to fend off a frontal attack. Sharks are best repulsed with blunt blows to the snout, eyes, or gills. If possible, do not use a bare hand. A stream of air bubbles from a scuba regulator directed into the face of a shark may be a sufficient deterrent. Although spears, knives, shotgun shell-loaded bang-stick powerheads, strychnine-filled spears, and carbon dioxide darts can kill small sharks, they can also worsen the situation if they are misapplied or if wounding a shark promotes a feeding frenzy within a school of animals.

BARRACUDA BITES

Barracuda bites should be managed in a fashion identical to that for shark bites.

BARRACUDA AVOIDANCE

Barracuda are attracted to turbid water, underwater commotion, irregular motion, surface splashing, shiny objects, and tethered fish. These should all be avoided. It is unwise to dangle a body part (e.g., ankle) adorned with reflective jewelry that simulates a lure before the jaws of a barracuda.

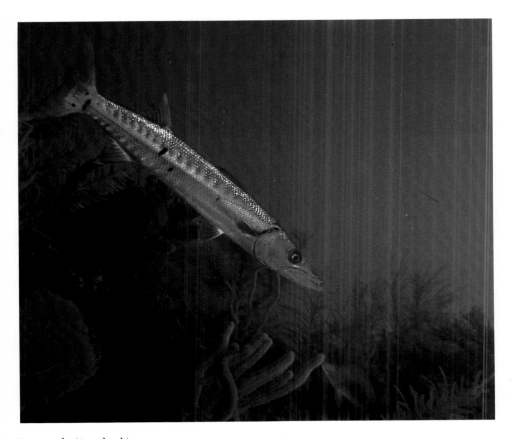

Barracuda (Auerbach)

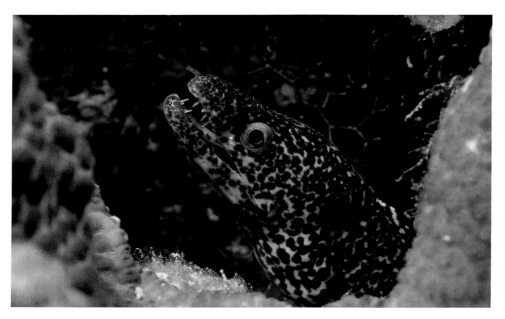

Moray eel (Auerbach)

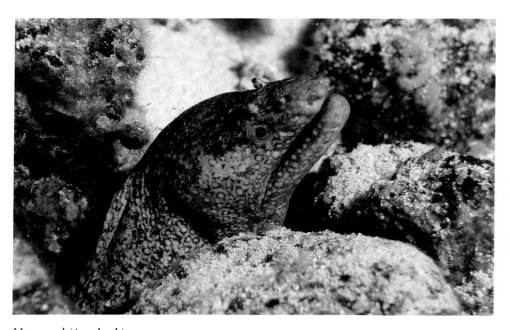

Moray eel (Auerbach)

MORAY EEL BITES

1. If the moray is still attached to the diver, pulling on the moray with extreme force is unlikely to detach the animal without breaking its teeth and leaving them in the wound or tearing the victim's flesh. To loosen the grip of the moray, it must be distracted or rendered unconscious. One technique is to offer the animal something more attractive to eat than the diver's arm, such as a bait fish. Unfortunately, this is rarely successful out of the water. If the animal cannot be coerced into letting go, it may need to be decapitated with a knife or have its jaw broken forcefully. *The animal should be injured as a last resort.*
2. Carefully clean the puncture wounds and remove all tooth fragments. Irrigate the wounds as best as is possible with disinfected (fresh) water with or without antiseptic solution (povidone-iodine 5% to 10%). Never close the small puncture wounds tightly with thread or tape. The risk of infection in such wounds, particularly of the hand and foot, is enormous.
3. If the wound shows signs of infection, administer antibiotics (see Marine Infections, p. 1). If a puncture wound is deep and on the hand or foot, administer antibiotics.

 ## NEEDLEFISH PUNCTURES

1. If the beak of a needlefish remains in the victim, gently slide the fish out of the victim. Manage the wound as you would a moray eel bite puncture. If the beak has penetrated *deeply* into the neck, head, chest, abdomen, or groin of the victim, do not remove it if you can bring the victim to a hospital within 24 hours. Break or cut the fish off gently 1 to 2 inches away from the body and pad and wrap the wound to prevent motion of the portion that remains in the victim. Seek immediate hospital attention. If you are more than 24 hours from formal medical care, carefully remove the fish (unless it is in the neck or head) and be prepared to manage brisk bleeding.
2. If the wound exhibits signs of infection, administer antibiotics (see Marine Infections, p. 1).

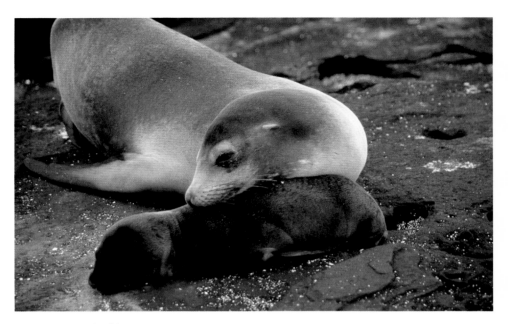

Sea lions (Auerbach)

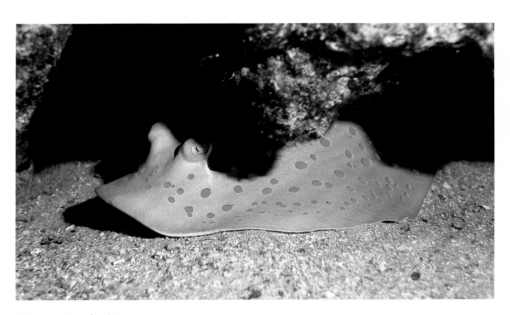

Stingray (Auerbach)

SEA LION BITES

Sea lions and seals are mild-mannered mammals, except during the mating season, at which time the males may become aggressive. During breeding season, both sexes will attack in defense of newborn pups. Divers have been seriously bitten, and therefore ill-tempered or overly aggressive animals should be avoided. Sea lion bites should be managed in a fashion identical to that for shark bites.

 ## TRIGGERFISH AND OTHER FISH BITES

All wounds incurred by fish teeth should be managed in a fashion identical to that for shark bites. If pain from the wound is out of proportion to the size of the injury, suspect an envenomation and treat the victim in the same manner described for a scorpionfish sting (see p. 17).

 ## STINGRAY ENVENOMATIONS

1. Rinse the wound vigorously with fresh water. Use ocean water only if fresh water is not immediately available.
2. Immerse the wound in nonscalding hot water to tolerance (110° to 113° F or 43.3° to 45° C) to achieve pain relief. This generally requires 30 to 90 minutes and may be repeated if pain recurs.
3. Remove any visible pieces of the stinger(s) or sheath. Scrub the wound with soap and water, then irrigate vigorously with fresh water.
4. Do not tape or sew the wound closed, unless this is necessary to stop excessive bleeding.
5. If the wound shows signs of infection, administer antibiotics (see Marine Infections, p. 1). If the wound is suspected to be deep (completely through the skin into fat or muscle), administer antibiotics.

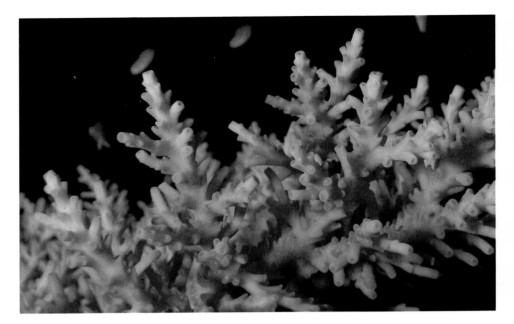

Coral (Auerbach)

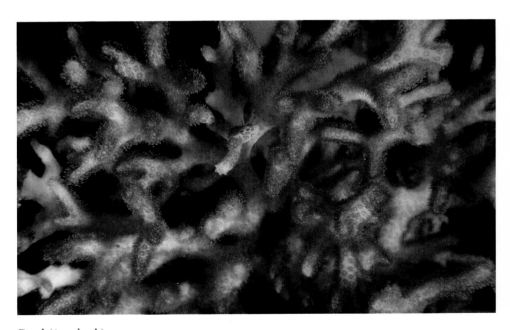

Coral (Auerbach)

CORAL AND BARNACLE CUTS

1. Scrub the cuts vigorously with soap and water, then flush the wounds with large amounts of fresh water or disinfected drinking water.
2. Flush the wound with a ½-strength solution of hydrogen peroxide in water to bubble out the "coral dust." Rinse again with fresh water.
3. Apply a thin layer of bacitracin ointment, and cover the wound loosely with a dry sterile dressing. If no ointment or dressing is available, the wound may be left open.
4. Scrub and rinse the wound twice a day. Reapply the ointment.
5. If the wound shows signs of infection, administer antibiotics (see Marine Infections, p. 1).

SCORPIONFISH (LIONFISH, ZEBRAFISH, STONEFISH) ENVENOMATIONS

1. Immerse the punctures in nonscalding hot water to tolerance (110° to 113° F or 43.3° to 45° C) to achieve pain relief. This generally requires 30 to 90 minutes and may be repeated if pain recurs.
2. Remove any visible pieces of the spine(s) or sheath. Scrub the wound with soap and water, then irrigate vigorously with fresh water.
3. Do not tape or sew the wound(s) closed.
4. If the wound shows signs of infection, administer antibiotics (see Marine Infections, p. 1). If a puncture wound is deep into the hand or foot, administer antibiotics.
5. In Australia (and other areas of the Indo-Pacific), an *antivenin* is available to physicians for treatment of the sting of the dreaded stonefish. Aquarists stung by captive stonefish in the United States can be treated with antivenin procured by a physician through a poison control center, zoo, or marine aquarium.

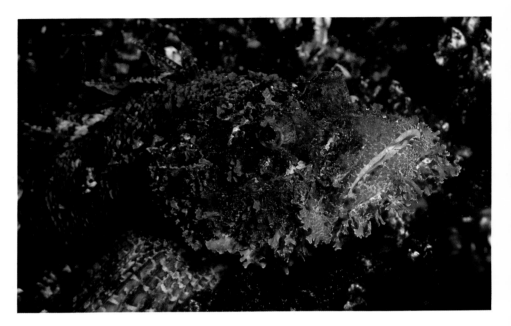

Scorpionfish (Auerbach)

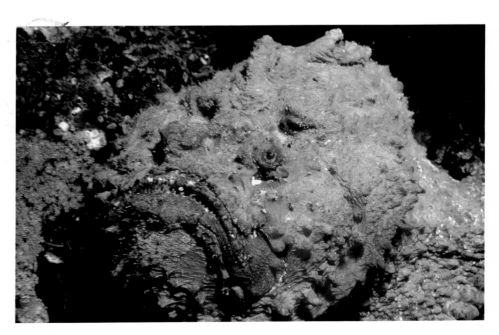

Stonefish (Roessler)

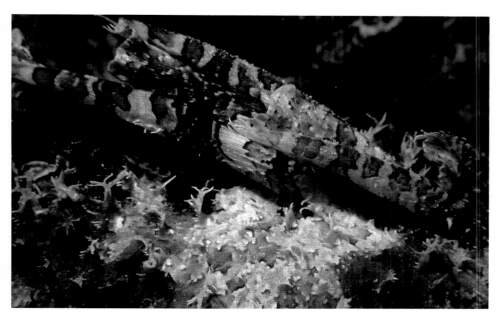

Scorpionfish spines (Kizer)

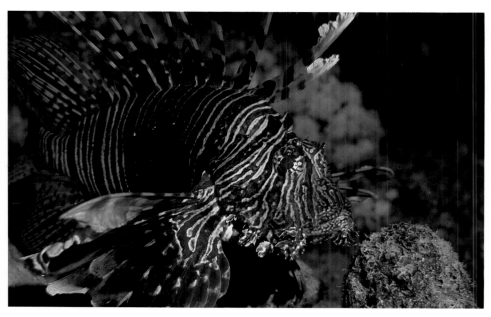

Lionfish (Auerbach)

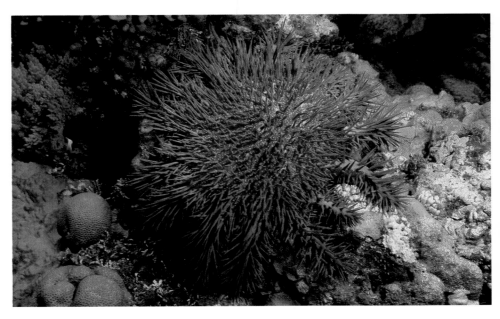

Crown-of-thorns starfish (Auerbach)

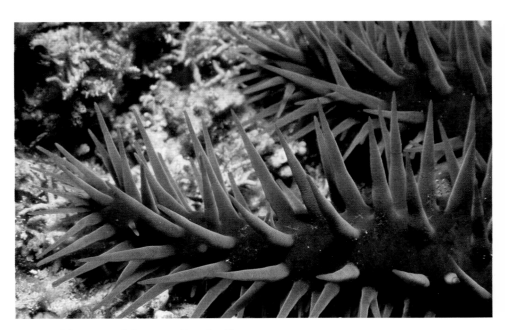

Crown-of-thorns starfish spines (Auerbach)

CATFISH STINGS

1. Immerse the puncture wounds in nonscalding hot water to tolerance (110° to 113° F or 43.3° to 45° C) to achieve pain relief. This generally requires 30 to 90 minutes and may be repeated if pain recurs.
2. Remove any visible pieces of the spine(s) or sheath. Scrub the wound with soap and water, then irrigate vigorously with fresh water.
3. Do not tape or sew the wound closed.
4. If the wound shows signs of infection, administer antibiotics (see Marine Infections, p. 1).

 ## WEEVERFISH STINGS

1. Immerse the puncture wounds in nonscalding hot water to tolerance (110° to 113° F or 43.3° to 45° C) to achieve pain relief. This generally requires 30 to 90 minutes and may be repeated if pain recurs.
2. Remove any visible pieces of the spine(s) or sheath. Scrub the wound with soap and water, then irrigate vigorously with fresh water.
3. Do not tape or sew the wound closed.
4. If the wound shows signs of infection, administer antibiotics (see Marine Infections, p. 1).

 ## STARFISH PUNCTURES

1. Immerse the puncture wounds in nonscalding hot water to tolerance (110° to 113° F or 43.3° to 45° C) to achieve pain relief. This generally requires 30 to 90 minutes and may be repeated if pain recurs.
2. Remove any visible pieces of the spine(s) or sheath. Scrub the wound with soap and water, then irrigate vigorously with fresh water.
3. Do not tape or sew the wound(s) closed.
4. If the wound shows signs of infection, administer antibiotics (see Marine Infections, p. 1).

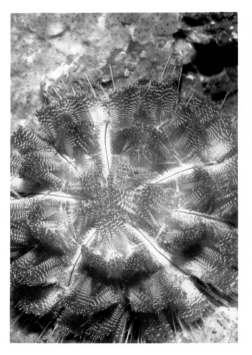

Urchin (Kizer)

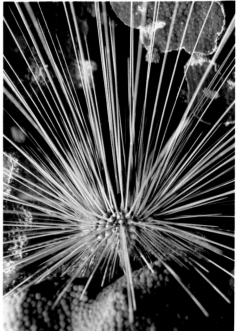

Urchin (Auerbach)

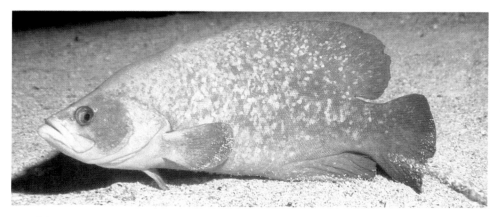

Soapfish (Roessler)

SEA URCHIN PUNCTURES

1. Immerse the puncture wounds in nonscalding hot water to tolerance (110° to 113° F or 43.3° to 45° C) to achieve pain relief. This generally requires 30 to 90 minutes and may be repeated if pain recurs.
2. Remove any visible pieces of the spine(s). This must be performed very gently to avoid breaking off any spines in the skin. Do not dig around in the skin to try to extract them; you will only crush the spines and make them more difficult to remove.
3. Purple or black discoloration of the skin at the puncture site does not necessarily mean that a spine is present. The "tattoo" may be dye leached from the surface of a spine that was withdrawn.
4. If a spine(s) has penetrated into or near a joint, it may need to be removed surgically so that there is no damage to nerves or important blood vessels. This should be accomplished by a physician as soon as possible to prevent the formation of scar tissue around the spine, which makes removal more difficult.
5. Do not crush a spine in the skin. Although smaller fragments may dissolve, this is not always the case, and you will make it nearly impossible to find all of the pieces.
6. If the urchin has envenomed with pedicellariae (pincers) rather than with spines, remove these by applying a lather of shaving cream or soap and then gently shaving the area. Hot water treatment may not be as effective in relieving the pain.
7. Scrub the wound(s) with soap and water, then irrigate vigorously with fresh water.
8. Do not tape or sew the wound(s) closed.
9. If the wound shows signs of infection, administer antibiotics (see Marine Infections, p. 1). If the puncture is deep into a hand or foot, administer antibiotics.

SOAPFISH IRRITATION

1. Wash the skin vigorously with soap and water.
2. Apply cool compresses, calamine lotion, or another soothing skin cream.
3. If swelling and itching persist beyond 24 hours, apply hydrocortisone

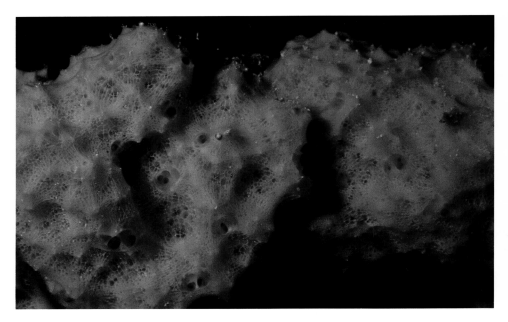

Orange sponge (Auerbach)

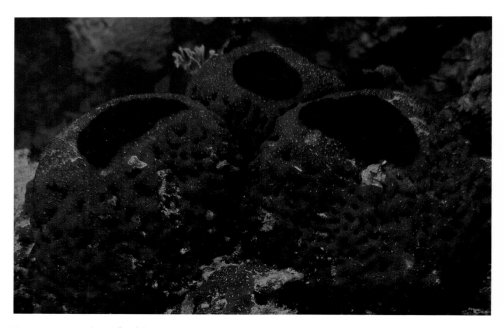

Brown sponge (Auerbach)

cream, ointment, or lotion (0.5% to 1%). If signs of infection appear, discontinue the use of any topical corticosteroid-containing preparation.
4. If swelling and itching are severe, administer an antihistamine and prednisone (see Allergic Reaction, p. 5).

 ## SEAWEED DERMATITIS

1. Scrub the skin vigorously with soap and water. Rinse with copious amounts of fresh water.
2. Rinse the affected skin with isopropyl alcohol (40% to 70%). Allow the skin to dry.
3. Apply a thin coating of hydrocortisone cream, ointment, or lotion (0.5% to 1%) twice a day. If signs of infection appear, discontinue the use of any topical corticosteroid-containing preparation.
4. If itching, blistering, and pain are severe, administer an antihistamine and prednisone (see Allergic Reaction, p. 5).
5. If the wound shows signs of infection, administer antibiotics (see Marine Infections, p. 1).

 ## SEA SPONGE IRRITATION

1. Soak the affected skin with 5% acetic acid (vinegar) for 10 to 15 minutes. This may be done by wetting a gauze pad or cloth with vinegar and applying it to skin. After soaking, dry the skin. If vinegar is not available, use isopropyl alcohol (40% to 70%) for 5 minutes. Dry the skin.
2. Apply the sticky side of adhesive tape to the skin and peel it off. This will remove most sponge spicules that protrude from the skin.
3. Repeat the vinegar soak for 5 minutes (or alcohol for 1 minute).
4. Apply a thin coating of hydrocortisone lotion (0.5% to 1%) twice a day until the irritation is gone. *Do not use hydrocortisone as the initial decontaminant before the application of vinegar or alcohol.*
5. If swelling, itching, blistering, and pain are severe, administer an antihistamine and prednisone (see Allergic Reaction, p. 5).
6. If the rash worsens and shows signs of infection (cloudy blisters, increasing redness or pain, swollen lymph glands, fever), administer antibiotics. Discontinue the use of any topical corticosteroid-containing preparation.

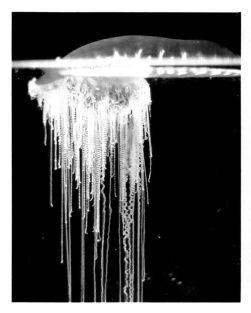

Man-of-war (Madin)

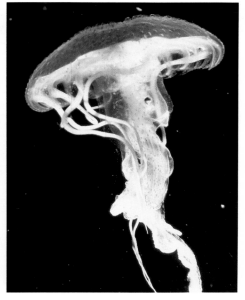

Mauve stinger jellyfish (Madin)

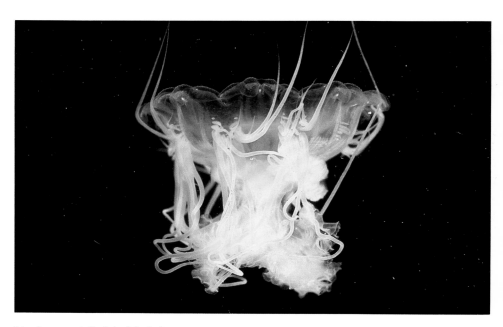

Lion's mane jellyfish (Madin)

JELLYFISH STINGS—INCLUDING MAN-OF-WAR, BOX JELLYFISH, SEA NETTLE, IRUKANDJI, ANEMONE, HYDROID

1. Immediately rinse the skin with sea water. *Do not rinse with fresh water. Do not apply ice. Do not rub the skin.*
2. Apply soaks of acetic acid 5% (vinegar) until the pain is relieved. If vinegar is not available, use isopropyl alcohol 40% to 70%. *In the case of the Australian box jellyfish, use vinegar in preference to alcohol.* If these are not available, briefly apply aluminum sulfate/surfactant (Stingose), dilute (¼ strength) ammonia, a paste of baking soda or unseasoned meat tenderizer, mashed papaya, or urine. Do not use methylated spirits (aftershave) or liquor for pain relief. *Do not apply organic solvents, such as kerosene, turpentine, or gasoline.* Do not apply meat tenderizer for longer than 10 minutes to the skin of children. A cold (ice) pack may be helpful, as long as there is no leak or surface condensation.

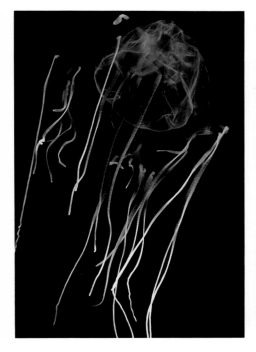

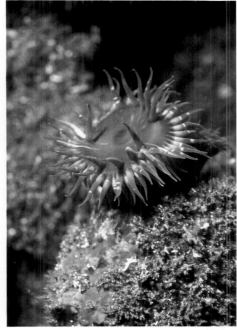

Box jellyfish (Keith Gillett: World Life
Research Institute)

Sea anemone (Auerbach)

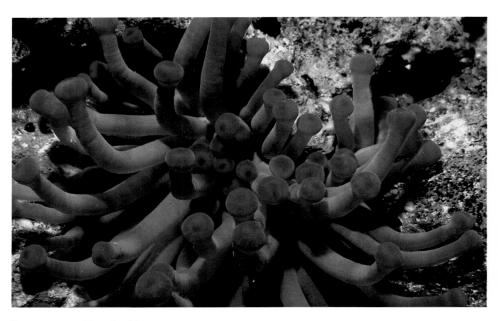

Sea anemone (Auerbach)

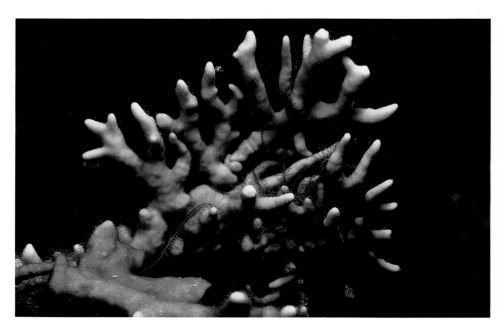

Fire coral (Auerbach)

3. Remove large tentacle fragments using forceps. Take care not to handle tentacles with bare hands. Wear gloves if possible when removing tentacles.

4. Apply a lather of shaving cream or a paste of baking soda (in an isolated area, you can use a paste of sand or mud in seawater), and shave the affected area with a razor or knife. If a razor is not available, use a sharp-edged object, such as a clamshell.

5. Reapply the vinegar or other decontaminant for 15 minutes.

6. Apply a thin coating of hydrocortisone lotion (0.5% to 1%) twice a day. If signs of an infection appear, discontinue the use of any corticosteroid-containing preparation.

7. If tentacle fragments are placed in the mouth (by a small child or intoxicated adult), immediately have the victim swish and spit whatever beverage is available. If there is already swelling in the mouth (muffled voice, difficulty swallowing, enlarged tongue and lips), do not give anything by mouth so that the victim does not choke.

8. If the eyes are stung by jellyfish, sea cucumbers, hydroid fragments, or other envenoming creatures, irrigate them with at least 1 to 2 liters (quarts) of fresh water. *Do not irrigate the eyes with vinegar, alcohol, or other decontaminant.*

 ## FIRE CORAL STINGS

1. Immediately rinse the skin **with sea water.** *Do not rinse with fresh water. Do not apply ice. Do not rub the skin.*

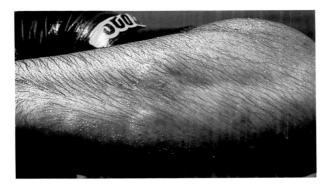

Fire coral sting (Kizer)

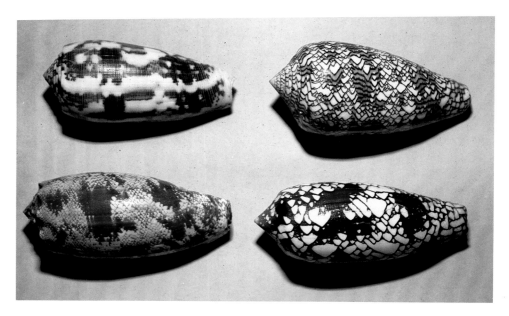

Cone shells (Auerbach)

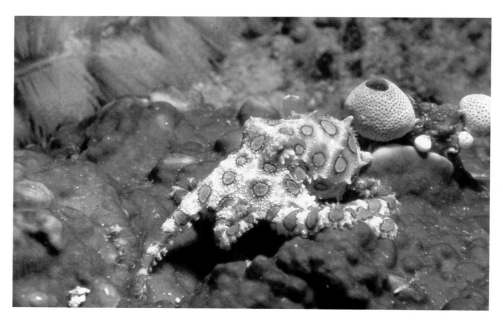

Blue-ringed octopus (Roessler)

2. Apply soaks of acetic acid 5% (vinegar) until the pain is relieved. If vinegar is unavailable, use isopropyl alcohol 40% to 70%. If these are not available, apply aluminum sulfate/surfactant (Stingose), dilute (¼-strength) ammonia, a paste of baking soda or unseasoned meat tenderizer, mashed papaya, or urine. Do not use methylated spirits (aftershave) or liquor for pain relief. *Do not apply organic solvents, such as kerosene, turpentine, or gasoline*. Do not apply meat tenderizer for longer than 10 minutes to the skin of children. A cold (ice) pack may be helpful, as long as there is no leak or surface condensation.
3. Apply a thin coating of hydrocortisone lotion (0.5% to 1%) twice a day. If signs of an infection appear, discontinue the use of any topical corticosteroid-containing preparation.

 ## CONE SHELL STINGS

1. If the sting occurs on the arm or leg, apply the "pressure-immobilization technique." Place a cloth or gauze pad of approximately 6 to 8 cm (length) × 6 to 8 cm (width) × 2 to 3 cm (thickness) directly over the sting. Hold it firmly in place by wrapping an elastic or cloth bandage around the bandage and limb, with margins of 2 to 3 cm above and below the pad. Wrap it tightly enough to press the pad into the skin but not so tight as to occlude the circulation (the victim's fingers or toes should remain pink and with normal sensation). Keep the bandage in place until the victim can be brought to a hospital. If evacuation is not possible, remove the bandage after 18 to 24 hours.
2. Bring the victim directly to a hospital.
3. Do not use incision and suction techniques. Do not apply a tourniquet.
4. Immersion into nonscalding hot water to tolerance (110° to 113° F or 43.3° to 45° C) may be of limited value to inactivate the venom and provide pain relief. It is no substitute for the pressure-immobilization technique.

 ## OCTOPUS BITES

1. If a sting from a blue-ringed octopus occurs on the arm or leg, apply the "pressure-immobilization technique." Place a cloth or gauze pad of approximately 6 to 8 cm (length) × 6 to 8 cm (width) × 2 to 3 cm (thickness) directly over the sting. Hold it firmly in place by wrapping an elastic cloth

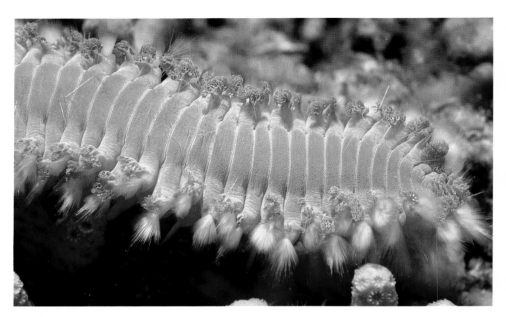

Bristleworm (Auerbach)

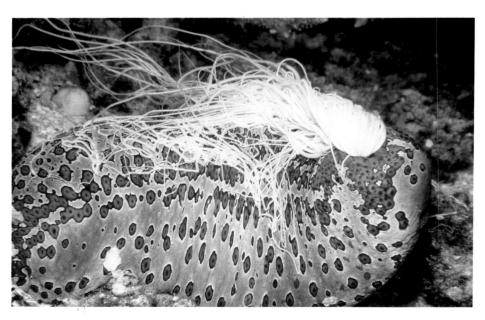

Sea cucumber with extended tentacles (Auerbach)

bandage around the bandage and limb, with margins of 2 to 3 cm above and below the pad. Wrap it tightly enough to press the pad into the skin, but not so tight as to occlude the circulation (the victim's fingers or toes should remain pink and with normal sensation). Keep the bandage in place until the victim can be brought to a hospital. If evacuation is not possible, remove the bandage after 18 to 24 hours.
2. Bring the victim directly to a hospital.
3. Do not use incision and suction techniques. Do not apply a tourniquet.
4. If the bite is from the Australian blue-ringed octopus, anticipate that the victim will become paralyzed and have difficulty breathing and may require artificial ventilation (respiration). The toxin (tetrodotoxin) is identical to that found in pufferfish.
5. Other octopus species are far less dangerous. Nontetrodotoxic octopus bites should receive the same wound care as do moray eel bites.

 ## BRISTLEWORM STINGS

1. All large visible bristles should be removed with forceps.
2. Dry the skin without scraping to avoid embedding the spines further into the skin.
3. Apply a layer of adhesive tape (sticky side to the skin) to remove the remaining smaller spines that are too tiny for individual extraction. Alternately, a "facial peel" may be applied and removed.
4. Apply acetic acid 5% (vinegar), isopropyl alcohol 40% to 70%, dilute ammonia, or a watery paste of unseasoned meat tenderizer (papain) to provide some pain relief.
5. If the reaction becomes severe, the victim may benefit from the application of topical corticosteroid-containing preparations.

 ## SEA CUCUMBER IRRITATIONS

1. Immediately rinse the skin **with sea water.** *Do not rinse with fresh water. Do not apply ice. Do not rub the skin.*
2. Apply soaks of acetic acid 5% (vinegar) until the pain is relieved. If vinegar is unavailable, use isopropyl alcohol 40% to 70%. If these are unavailable, apply aluminum sulfate/surfactant (Stingose), dilute (¼-strength) ammo-

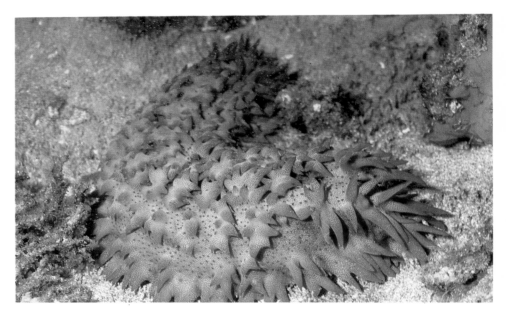

Sea cucumber (Auerbach)

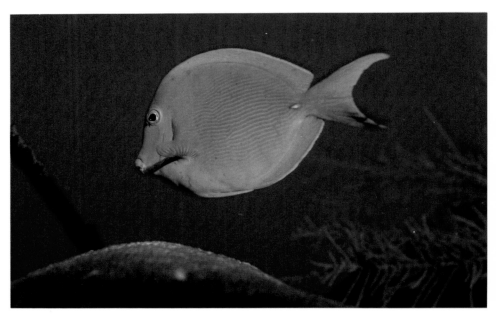

Surgeonfish (Auerbach)

nia, a paste of baking soda or unseasoned meat tenderizer, mashed papaya, or urine. Do not rely on methylated spirits (aftershave) or liquor for pain relief. *Do not apply organic solvents, such as kerosene, turpentine, or gasoline.* Do not apply meat tenderizer for longer than 10 minutes to the skin of children.
3. If the eyes are irritated, irrigate them with at least 1 to 2 L of fresh water. *Do not rinse the eyes with vinegar, alcohol, or other decontaminant.*

 ## ANNELID WORM BITES

1. Apply soaks of acetic acid 5% (vinegar) until the pain is relieved. If vinegar is unavailable, use isopropyl alcohol 40% to 70%. If these are unavailable, apply aluminum sulfate/surfactant (Stingose), dilute (¼-strength) ammonia, a paste of baking soda or unseasoned meat tenderizer, mashed papaya, or urine. Do not apply meat tenderizer for longer than 10 minutes to the skin of children.

 ## SURGEONFISH CUTS

1. Immerse the punctures in nonscalding hot water to tolerance (110° to 113° F or 43.3° to 45° C) to achieve pain relief. This generally requires 30 to 90 minutes and may be repeated if pain recurs.
2. Remove any visible pieces of the blade or sheath. Scrub the wound with soap and water, then irrigate vigorously with fresh water.
3. Do not tape or sew the wound closed.

 ## SEA SNAKE BITES

1. If the sting occurs on the arm or leg, apply the "pressure-immobilization technique." Place a cloth or gauze pad of approximately 6 to 8 cm (length) × 6 to 8 cm (width) × 2 to 3 cm (thickness) directly over the sting. Hold it firmly in place by wrapping an elastic or cloth bandage around the bandage and limb, with margins of 2 to 3 cm above and below the pad.

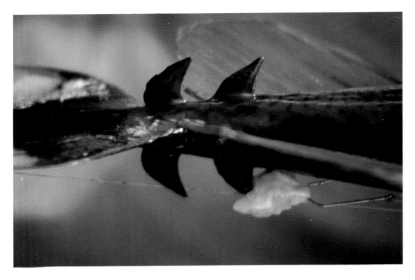

Surgeonfish blades (Auerbach)

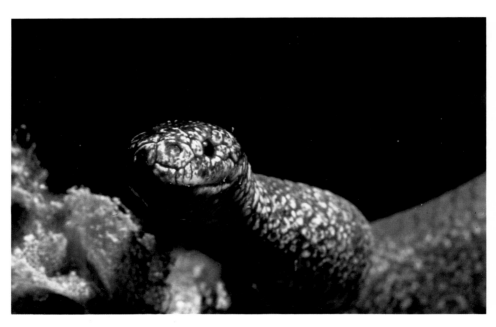

Sea snake (Roessler)

Wrap it tightly enough to press the pad into the skin, but not so tight as to occlude the circulation (the victim's fingers or toes should remain pink and with normal sensation). Keep the bandage in place until the victim can be brought to a hospital. If no symptoms develop and evacuation is not possible, remove the bandage after 18 to 24 hours.

2. Bring the victim directly to a hospital. *The definitive treatment is the administration of antivenin.*

3. Do not use incision and suction techniques. Do not apply a tourniquet. Do not apply ice directly to the wound. Use a commercial suction device (The Extractor) *if it can be applied within 5 minutes of the bite.* Otherwise (or after suction), apply the pressure-immobilization technique.

4. If the victim does not develop symptoms within 6 to 8 hours, it is unlikely that a significant poisoning has occurred. Symptoms include weakness, paralysis, lockjaw, drooping eyelids, blurred vision, difficulty speaking and swallowing, and vomiting. If mild symptoms develop following pressure-immobilization of the wound, do not release the bandage until the victim can be brought to a medical center, even if there will be a prolonged delay. Early release of the bandage may allow a dangerous amount of venom to enter the victim's bloodstream, with disastrous effects.

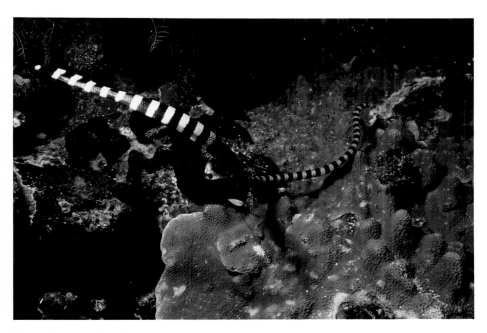

Sea snake (Auerbach)

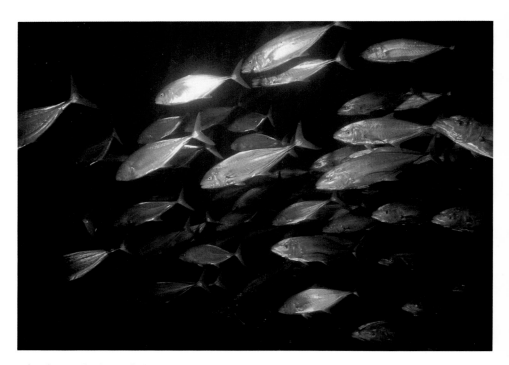

Schooling jacks (Roessler)

 FISH POISONINGS

A biological marine hazard is present in marine animals that are poisonous to eat. Many creatures are always poisonous, and hosts of others are toxic during certain seasons of the year, usually in relation to reproductive cycles. These include dinoflagellates, coelenterates, mollusks, echinoderms, crustaceans, fishes, turtles, and mammals. Whenever a person develops an unexplained illness during or following a diving trip, it is important to have an appropriate index of suspicion for poisoning and to obtain an accurate dietary history. Only in this manner can you reach a proper diagnosis. This is very important, as rapid and appropriate treatment may be lifesaving.

Marine biotoxins are most commonly natural poisons derived directly from marine organisms. These include phytotoxins (plant poisonings) or zootoxins (animal poisonings). With regard to fish and shellfish, some toxins are produced directly by the animal, whereas others are concentrated within the animal as it dines on smaller creatures and absorbs poisons that have been created lower in the food chain.

Never rely on cooking or soaking (leaching) techniques to destroy or remove toxins from fish or shellfish. This is fraught with hazard and often results in severe poisonings. Do not expect tainted seafood to have altered taste, odor, or color; frequently, the food appears normal in all respects. Trust the advice of local inhabitants when they caution you to avoid specific marine food products.

SCOMBROID POISONING

Scombroid fish include the albacore, bluefish, bluefin and yellowfin tuna, mackerel, saury, needlefish, wahoo, skipjack, and bonito. Nonscombroid fish that produce scombroid (mackerel-like) poisoning include mahi-mahi (dolphin), kahawai, sardine, anchovy, herring, amberjack (yellowtail or kahala), and the Australian ocean salmon.

During conditions of inadequate preservation or refrigeration, the muscles of these dark- or red-fleshed fish undergo bacterial decomposition, producing the chemical histamine. This and other toxins are heat and acid stable and are not destroyed by domestic or commercial cooking.

Affected fish often have a sharply metallic or peppery taste; however, they may be normal in appearance, color, and flavor. Not all persons who eat a contaminated fish may become ill, as the toxins may be unevenly distributed in a single fish.

Symptoms occur within 15 to 90 (usually less than 60) minutes of ingestion. These may include flushing (worsened with sun exposure and particularly of the face, neck, and upper torso), a sensation of warmth without elevated temperature, red eyes, itching, hives, puffy face and hands, difficulty breathing with wheezing, nausea, vomiting, diarrhea, upper abdominal burning (heartburn), lower abdominal cramps, difficulty swallowing, headache, thirst, sore throat, irritated gums, rapid and fluttering heartbeat, dizziness, and a low blood pressure level (shock). Untreated, a mild reaction generally resolves within 8 to 12 hours. Death is unusual.

Treatment

1. If the reaction is severe, manage it as you would an allergic reaction (p. 5).
2. For a *mild reaction* (with flushing, nausea, vomiting, diarrhea, itching, or slight shortness of breath), administer diphenhydramine (Benadryl). The adult dose is 25 to 50 mg every 4 to 6 hours; the child's dose is 1 mg/kg.

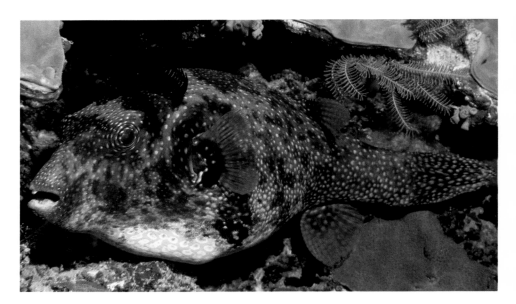

Pufferfish (Roessler)

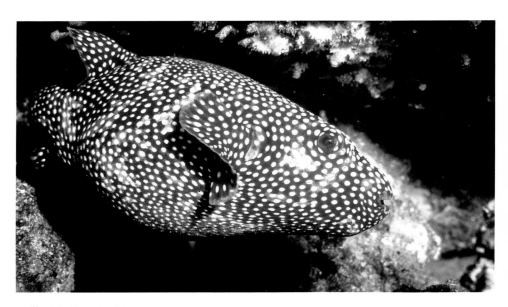

Pufferfish (Auerbach)

Two alternative drugs are cimetidine (Tagamet) in an adult dose of 300 mg every 6 to 8 hours or ranitidine (Zantac) 150 mg every 12 hours.

3. If a large amount of the fish has been consumed within the previous hour, it may help to induce vomiting. This should only be done if the victim is not having any difficulty breathing. Often, the victim will vomit spontaneously, so this is unnecessary.

4. For a *severe or prolonged reaction*, seek immediate attention. For persistent headache, effective drugs include cimetidine (Tagamet) in an adult dose of 300 mg by mouth every 6 to 8 hours, ranitidine (Zantac) 150 mg every 12 hours, or acetaminophen (Tylenol) in an adult dose of 650 mg by mouth every 6 to 8 hours.

Prevention

Scombroid poisoning can be avoided to a certain extent with proper refrigeration of fish. All captured fish should be gutted, cooled, and placed on ice immediately. No fish should be consumed if it has been handled improperly, has the smell of ammonia, or an abnormal taste. Fresh fish generally have a sheen or oily rainbow appearance; dull-appearing fish should be avoided.

TETRODOTOXIN (PUFFERFISH) POISONING

Tetrodotoxin is one of the most potent nonprotein poisons found in nature. Tetrodotoxic fishes include pufferfish (toadfish, blowfish, globefish, swellfish, balloonfish, toado), sunfish, and porcupine fish. These are tropical and subtropical fish, some of which are prepared as delicacies *(fugu)* in Japan by specially trained and licensed chefs. The toxin is distributed throughout the entire fish, with the greatest concentrations in the liver, gonads (ovaries), intestine, and skin and lesser amounts in the muscles and blood.

The onset of symptoms can be as rapid as 10 minutes or can be delayed for up to 4 hours. Initially, victims develop oral numbness and tingling, with rapid progression to light-headedness and generalized numbness and tingling. The following symptoms develop rapidly: drooling, difficulty swallowing, sweating, fatigue, headache, nausea, vomiting, diarrhea, abdominal pain, weakness, difficulty speaking and walking, incoordination, uncontrollable shaking, paralysis, seizures, shortness of breath and difficulty breathing, coma, and a low blood pressure level (shock). Nausea and vomiting are often quite severe. Weakness and paralysis may first develop in the arms and descend to the legs. Sixty percent of victims will die, most of these within the first 6 hours.

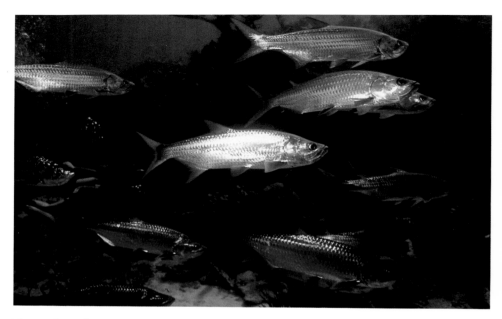

Tarpon (Roessler)

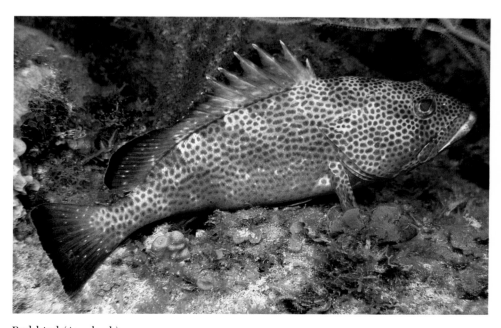

Red hind (Auerbach)

Treatment

1. Induce vomiting if the victim has eaten the toxic fish within the past 3 hours. *This should only be done if the victim is awake, alert, and not having any difficulty swallowing or breathing.* Do not induce further vomiting if the victim has already vomited.
2. If the victim is short of breath or unconscious, assist with breathing (artificial respiration). If the victim vomits, rapidly turn him on his side and clear out his mouth so that he does not inhale stomach contents. Remember that the paralyzed victim may be fully conscious (so long as he is breathing or you are breathing for him), so take care to offer verbal explanations and reassurances.
3. As soon as it is suspected that someone has eaten a toxic pufferfish, *seek immediate medical attention.*

Prevention

Although the toxin is water soluble, it is very difficult to remove from the fish, even by cooking. It is wisest to avoid all puffers, even when prepared by an expert.

CIGUATERA TOXIN POISONING

Ciguatoxin derives its name from *cigua*, the word Spanish settlers used to describe poisoning from ingestion of the poisonous marine turban shell snail found in the Caribbean Spanish Antilles. It involves tropical and semitropical marine coral reef fish, which feed on certain plants or bottom fish, implicating specific species of algae. As the fish within the food chain become larger, the toxin is accumulated, rendering larger (greater than 6 pounds) and elderly fish more toxic. Although the entire fish is toxic, the internal organs (particularly the liver) and roe carry the highest concentrations of toxin.

More than 400 species of fish have been implicated, with the greatest concentration in the Caribbean Sea, in the Pacific Ocean around the Indo-Pacific Islands, and along the continental tropical reefs. The most frequently implicated reef fishes include the moray eels, mullets, groupers, snappers, porgies, jacks, wrasses, parrotfishes, surgeonfishes, triggerfishes, and barracuda. More than 75% of reported cases (except in Hawaii) involve the barracuda, snapper, jack, or grouper. Other fishes that have been reported as ciguatoxic include ladyfishes, milkfishes, herrings, tarpon, anchovies, lizardfishes, true eels, snake eels, needlefishes, flying fishes, halfbeaks, trumpetfishes, seahorses, squirrelfishes, cardinalfishes, sea perches, butterfly fishes, hawkfishes, dolphins, oilfishes, silverfishes, gobies, sailfishes, bass,

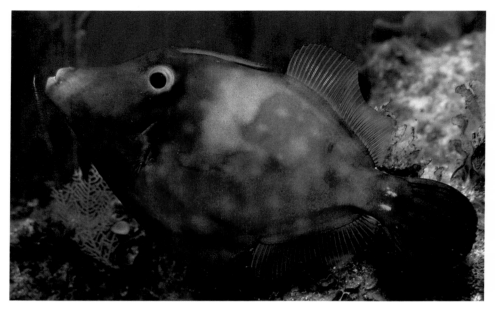

Filefish (Auerbach)

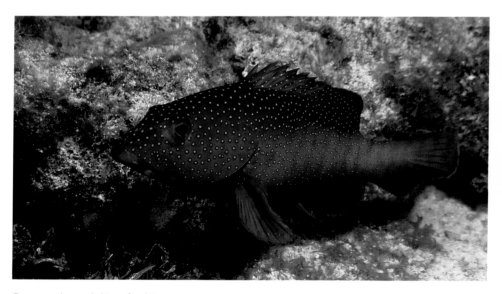

Grouper (coney) (Auerbach)

rudderfishes, goatfishes, sweeperfishes, damselfishes, grunts, spade fishes, croakers, tunas, scorpionfish, rabbitfishes, swordfishes, moorish idol, flounders, filefishes, trunkfishes, toadfishes, sargassumfish, goosefish, and longnose batfish.

All toxins identified to date are unaffected by freeze-drying, heat, cold, and stomach acid and do not affect the odor, color, or taste of the fish.

The onset of symptoms may be within 15 to 30 minutes of ingestion, is generally within 1 to 3 hours of ingestion, and shows an increase in severity over the ensuing 4 to 6 hours. Most victims have an onset of symptoms within 12 hours of ingestion and virtually all are afflicted within 24 hours. Symptoms include abdominal pain, nausea, vomiting, diarrhea, chills, numbness and tingling (particularly of the arms and legs and the area around the mouth), itching (usually of the palms and soles after a delay of 2 to 5 days), tongue and throat numbness or burning, sensation of "carbonation" during swallowing, fatigue, muscle quivering, stiff neck, dizziness, clumsy walking, pain and weakness in the legs, blurred vision, blindness, seizures, red and irritated eyes, red skin rash, blisters, drooling, sweating, headache, muscle and joint aches (particularly in the lower back and thighs), insomnia, abnormal heart rhythms, a low blood pressure level, coma, and difficulty breathing. More severe reactions tend to occur in persons who have been previously stricken with the disease. A classic symptom is the reversal of hot and cold perception, which develops in some persons after 3 to 5 days and may last for months.

Treatment

1. Induce vomiting if the victim has eaten the toxic fish within the past 3 hours. *This should only be done if the victim is awake, alert, and not having any difficulty swallowing or breathing.* Do not induce further vomiting if the victim has already vomited.
2. Save a piece of the fish for analysis. Preferably, freeze the sample.
3. Seek immediate medical attention.
4. In a mild case, cool showers or the administration of diphenhydramine (Benadryl) may help to relieve itching. The adult dose of Benadryl is 25 to 50 mg every 4 to 6 hours; the child's dose is 1 mg/kg. Moderate headache may be treated with acetaminophen (Tylenol).
5. After an episode of ciguatera poisoning, a victim should exclude the following from his diet: potentially ciguatera-toxic fish (fresh or preserved), fish sauces, shellfish, shellfish sauces, alcoholic beverages, nuts, and nut oils.

Prevention

Because of the accumulation of toxin, all oversized fish of any likely predaceous reef species (e.g., jack, snapper, barracuda, grouper, or parrot-beaked bottom feeder) should be suspected. The internal organs of tropical marine fish should be discarded. Moray eels should never be eaten. If it is necessary to eat fish in a survival situation, a small portion of the fish in question may be fed to a sacrificial small animal, which is then observed for ill effects for 12 hours. *Unreliable tests* that have been popularized in folklore include: a lone fish (separated from the school) should not be eaten; ants and turtles refuse to eat ciguatoxic fish; if a thin slice does not show a rainbow effect when held up to the sun it is ciguatoxic; and a silver spoon tarnishes in a cooking pot with ciguatoxic fish.

CLUPEOTOXIN POISONING

Clupeotoxic fish poisoning can occur when plankton-feeding fish are consumed. These fish are found in tropical Caribbean, Indo-Pacific, and African coastal waters. Examples include herrings, sardines, anchovies, tarpons, bonefishes, and deep-sea slickheads. Toxicity is reported to increase during the warm summer months. The internal organs are often highly toxic.

The onset of symptoms is rapid and characterized as "violent," often within 30 to 60 minutes of ingestion and rarely delayed beyond 2 hours. These include a marked metallic taste, dry mouth, nausea, vomiting, diarrhea, and abdominal pain. These are followed by chills, headache, sweating, severe numbness and tingling, muscle cramps, dizziness, fatigue, rapid heartbeat, blue discoloration of the fingers, lips, nose, toes or a combination of these (similar to that seen with exposure to cold temperatures), a low blood pressure level (shock), and death in up to 45% of cases. As with ciguatera toxin, the poison does not impart any unusual appearance, odor, or flavor to the fish.

Treatment

1. Induce vomiting if the victim has eaten the toxic fish within the past 3 hours. *This should only be done if the victim is awake, alert, and not having any difficulty swallowing or breathing.* Do not induce further vomiting if the victim has already vomited.
2. Seek immediate medical attention. The poisoning is so unusual and so rarely suspected (because of a lack of clues as to the cause) that this is not often carried out. Aggressive hospital management and early intensive care are essential.

Prevention

Clupeotoxic fish should be avoided, especially during summer months, in fish indigenous to the Caribbean, African coastal, or Indo-Pacific waters.

PARALYTIC SHELLFISH POISONING

Shellfish filter large quantities of water to gather plankton and extract oxygen, which allows for a concentration of bacteria, viruses, and biological toxins.

Paralytic shellfish poisoning (PSP) is induced by ingesting any of a variety of filter-feeding organisms. These include familiar mollusks (e.g., clams, oysters, scallops, and mussels), chitons, limpets, murex, starfish, reef crabs, and sandcrabs. They accumulate and concentrate biological toxins by feeding on various planktons and protozoans. These microorganisms prefer warm and sunlit water in which to "bloom," causing "red" and other-colored "tides." Outbreaks of shellfish poisoning have been reported in North America, Europe, Africa, Asia, and the Pacific islands, with the latter linked to certain Pacific crabs and lobsters.

In shellfish, the greatest concentrations of toxin (saxitoxin) are found in the digestive organs, gills, and siphon. However, there is no physical characteristic that distinguishes the carrier animal. The toxin is water-soluble, heat-stable, and stomach acid-stable. Like tetrodotoxin, it is not destroyed by ordinary cooking.

Within minutes to a few hours of ingestion of contaminated shellfish, there is the onset of numbness and tingling inside and around the mouth, notably of the tongue and gums. These symptoms progress rapidly to involve the neck, hands, and feet. Other symptoms rapidly develop, including light-headedness, loss of balance, incoordination, weakness, difficulty speaking and swallowing, drooling, thirst, diarrhea, abdominal pain, nausea, vomiting, blurred vision, headache, sweating, a sensation of loose teeth, chest pain, and rapid heartbeat. Paralysis and respiratory insufficiency may follow. If the victim can breathe or if you are breathing for him, the victim will often remain awake and alert, although paralyzed. Up to 25% of victims expire from respiratory failure within the first 12 hours.

Treatment

1. Induce vomiting if the victim has eaten toxic fish within the past 3 hours. *This should only be done if the victim is awake, alert, and not having any*

difficulty swallowing or breathing. Do not induce further vomiting if the victim has already vomited.

2. The greatest danger is respiratory paralysis. *If the victim is short of breath or unconscious,* assist breathing (artificial respiration). If the victim vomits, rapidly turn him on his side and clear out his mouth so that he does not inhale stomach contents. Remember that the paralyzed victim may be fully conscious (so long as he is breathing or you are breathing for him), so take care to offer verbal explanations and reassurances.

3. As soon as it is suspected that someone has eaten a toxic shellfish, *seek immediate medical attention.* Do not allow the victim to consume alcoholic beverages.

Prevention

Although leaching of shellfish in fresh water for several weeks, followed by vigorous cooking, may remove up to 70% of the toxin, such procedures are recommended only for persons stranded on desert islands. To the old axiom "don't eat shellfish in the Northern hemisphere in months that contain the letter *r*" should be added "it doesn't matter how you spell the month if the shellfish are contaminated with saxitoxin."

HALLUCINATORY FISH POISONING

Fish that cause hallucinatory fish poisoning are predominantly reef fish of the tropical Pacific and Indian Ocean reefs, which carry the toxins in the head parts, brain, and spinal cord, with lesser amounts of poison in the flesh. Typical species include surgeonfish, chub, mullet, unicornfish, goatfish, sergeant major, grouper, rabbitfish, rock cod, drumfish, rudderfish, and damselfish.

Symptoms develop within 5 to 90 minutes of ingestion and include dizziness, numbness and tingling of the mouth and throat, sore throat, sweating, weakness, incoordination, hallucinations, nightmares, depression, shortness of breath, and slight paralysis.

Treatment

1. Induce vomiting if the victim has eaten the toxic fish within the past 3 hours. *This should only be done if the victim is awake, alert, and not having any difficulty swallowing or breathing.* Do not induce further vomiting if the victim has already vomited.

2. Seek immediate medical attention.

3. If the victim is agitated or violent, keep him from doing anything fool-
   ish or from harming bystanders. Observe the victim until he is clearly
   normal.

Prevention

Do not eat the head, brain, or spinal cord of any tropical fish. Heat does
not inactivate the toxin.

FISH LIVER POISONING

A fish may carry potent toxins in its liver. The remainder of the fish may
be nontoxic. There is some evidence to suggest that the toxic principle is
Vitamin A. Fish that are always toxic include Japanese perchlike fish (e.g.,
mackerel, sea bass, porgy, and sandfish) and tropical sharks (e.g., requiem,
sleeper, cow, great white, cat, hammerhead, angel, Greenland, and dogfish).
In addition, some skates and rays carry toxins in the liver.

Ingestion of the Japanese perchlike fish causes symptoms within the first
hour, with maximum intensity over the ensuing 6 hours. Symptoms include
nausea, vomiting, headache, skin flushing, rash, fever, and rapid heartbeat.
Ingestion of the toxic shark liver also causes symptoms in the first 30 to
60 minutes, which include nausea, vomiting, diarrhea, abdominal pain,
weakness, sweating, headache, sore mouth and throat, muscle cramps,
sore joints, numbness and tingling, hiccoughs, loss of balance, involuntary
urination, blurred vision, agitation, difficulty breathing, coma, and rarely,
death.

Treatment

1. Induce vomiting if the victim has eaten the toxic fish within the past 3
   hours. *This should only be done if the victim is awake, alert, and not
   having any difficulty swallowing or breathing.* Do not induce further
   vomiting if the victim has already vomited.
2. Seek immediate medical attention.

Prevention

1. Never eat the liver of any fish or other form of marine life. Do not eat
   any internal organs from sharks. Dried shark flesh (muscle) may be
   somewhat safer, but this should not be regarded as an absolute protection.

ANEMONE POISONING

In the South Pacific, ingestion of certain green or brown anemones has been associated with severe illness and death. The toxic substances are found in the tentacles and their associated stingers.

Ingestion of a toxic raw anemone causes agitation within 30 minutes. The victim becomes confused, delirious, and then unconscious. Other symptoms include fever, seizures, muscle aching, abdominal pain, difficulty breathing, and a low blood pressure level. If the anemone touches the skin, particularly the sensitive tissue inside the mouth, there can be blistering.

Treatment

1. Unfortunately, the symptoms occur so rapidly that there is little that can be done to help the victim. Induce vomiting if the victim has eaten the toxic fish within the past 3 hours. *This should only be done if the victim is awake, alert, and not having any difficulty swallowing or breathing.* Do not induce further vomiting if the victim has already vomited.
2. Seek immediate medical attention. Be prepared for the victim's condition to become life-threatening.

AFFLICTIONS FROM EATING RAW FISH

There is an increasing popularity worldwide in the consumption of raw fish (*sushi* or *sashimi*), which has led to more frequent infestation with the fish tapeworm. Raw salmon is a popular culprit and should not be eaten unless it has first been completely frozen at an extremely low temperature.

Symptoms of fish tapeworm infestation include abdominal pain, nausea, vomiting, diarrhea, and weight loss. Worm segments may be passed in the stool. Chronic infestation causes anemia. The diagnosis is made by examining the stool under a microscope for typical worm segment or egg forms. Effective drug treatment can be prescribed by a physician.

Another hazard is anisakiasis, which is caused by penetration of nematode larvae through the lining of the stomach. These are ingested in mackerel, bream, squid, sardines, bonito, Pacific herring, sablefish, Pacific cod, arrowtooth flounder, petrale sole, coho salmon, Pacific ocean perch, silvergray rockfish, yellowtail rockfish, and boccaccio.

Symptoms begin within 1 hour of ingestion of the raw fish and include severe upper abdominal pain resembling heartburn, nausea, and vomiting. The worms may be coughed up, vomited, or excreted in the stool. The only effective treatment is physical removal of the worms from the gastrointestinal tract by a properly trained physician.

Prevention

Only eat cooked (above 60° C) or previously frozen (to −20° C) fish. Smoking, marinating, pickling, brining, and salting may not kill parasites. Because the egg forms and larvae are so small, candling and superficial inspection are not sufficient to detect the infestation. Fish should be gutted as soon as possible after they are caught to limit the migration of worms from the internal organs into the flesh.

VIBRIO FISH POISONING

Vibrios are bacteria that reside in the marine environment, particularly in the tissue of shellfish such as oysters, crawfish, and perhaps crab or shrimp. If persons eat contaminated animals, particularly raw, they may become infected and suffer from severe nausea, vomiting, diarrhea, fever, and dehydration. In addition, the infection can spread into the bloodstream of persons who suffer from altered immunity, such as those with alcoholism, diabetes, AIDS, or liver disease or those taking steroid medications regularly. When this occurs, a person can rapidly become overwhelmed and expire.

Treatment

Treatment is the administration of antibiotics by a physician. Any person who is stricken following the ingestion of raw shellfish should seek immediate medical care. If a physician is unavailable and the victim can keep liquids down, administer ciprofloxacin (500 to 750 mg) or trimethoprim-sulfamethoxazole double-strength twice a day for 3 to 4 days.

VIRAL (GASTROENTERIC) SHELLFISH POISONING

Bacterial and viral gastrointestinal diseases may be caused by the consumption of contaminated shellfish, particularly raw clams and oysters, dried and salted raw fish, crabs, shrimp, or home-preserved fish products. Steamed shellfish also pose a significant risk, as household cooking techniques are often insufficient to kill viruses.

The most common symptoms are diarrhea, abdominal cramps, nausea, vomiting, and fever. The incubation period is usually 24 to 48 hours, with a similar duration of symptoms in a self-limited illness.

Treatment

1. Dehydration is the major problem. Encourage the victim to drink clear fluids such as commercial electrolyte-enhanced beverages, club soda, and broth. Avoid milk-containing beverages and acidic fruit juices for 48 hours.
2. If vomiting is persistent and severe or the victim becomes severely dehydrated, seek immediate medical attention.

Prevention

There is clearly a risk associated with eating raw shellfish. Be certain that they have been harvested from clean waters or provided by a reputable source. Do not eat any shellfish that have a tainted odor or taste.

OTHER POISONINGS

A variety of other marine animals can cause human poisoning or parasite infestation. As a reminder, all of the following should be strictly avoided: polar bear liver, shark liver, castor oil fish, unfamiliar sea anemones, giant Tridacna clams, whelks, ivory shells, grass carp gall bladder, unfamiliar tropical crabs, raw ocean salmon or mackerel, and unfamiliar Indo-Pacific marine turtles.

 SUGGESTED READINGS

Acott C: Sea snake bites. S Pac Undersea Med Soc J 15:11, 1985.

Auerbach PS et al: Bacteriology of the marine environment: implications for clinical therapy. Ann Emerg Med 16:643-649, 1987.

Auerbach PS: Natural microbiologic hazards of the aquatic environment. Clin Dermatol 5(3):52-61, 1987.

Auerbach PS: Stings of the deep. Emerg Med 21:26-41, 1989.

Auerbach PS and Halstead BW: Hazardous aquatic life. In Auerbach PS and Geehr EC, editors: Management of wilderness and environmental emergencies. St Louis, 1989, The CV Mosby Co., pp. 933-1028.

Blake PA: Vibrios on the half shell: what the walrus and the carpenter didn't know. Ann Intern Med 99:558-559, 1983.

Buck JD, Spotte S, and Gadbaw JJ: Bacteriology of the teeth from a great white shark: potential medical implications for shark bite victims. J Clin Microbiol 20:849-851, 1984.

Burnett JW, Rubinstein H, and Calton GJ: First aid for jellyfish envenomation. South Med J 76:870-872, 1983.

Fenner PJ et al: The "Irukandji" syndrome and acute pulmonary oedema. Med J Aust 149:150-156, 1988.

Fenner PJ, Williamson JA, and Skinner RA: Fatal and non-fatal stingray envenomation. Med J Aust 151:621-625, 1989.

Fenner PJ, Williamson JA, and Blenkin JA: Successful use of *Chironex* antivenom by members of the Queenland Ambulance Transport Brigade. Med J Aust 151:708-710, 1989.

Halstead BW: Poisonous and venomous marine animals of the world, ed 2. Princeton, 1988, The Darwin Press, Inc.

Halstead BW, Auerbach PS, and Campbell D: A colour atlas of dangerous marine animals. London, 1990, Wolfe Medical Publications Ltd.

Kizer KW, McKinney HE, and Auerbach PS: Scorpaenidae envenomation: a five-year poison center experience. JAMA 253:807-810, 1985.

Kliks MM: Human anisakiasis: an update. JAMA 255:2605, 1986 (editorial).

Maretic Z and Russell FE: Stings by the sea anemone *Anemonia sulcata* in the Adriatic Sea. Am J Trop Med Hyg 32:891-896, 1983.

Palafox NA et al: Successful treatment of ciguatera fish poisoning with intravenous mannitol. JAMA 259:2740-2742, 1988.

Pien FD et al: Bacterial flora of marine penetrating injuries. Diagn Microbiol Infect Dis 1:229-232, 1983.

Ragelis EP, editor: Seafood toxins. Washington, DC, 1984, The American Chemical Society.

Sims JK and Ostman DC: Pufferfish poisoning: emergency diagnosis and management of mild human tetrodotoxication. Ann Emerg Med 15:1094-1098, 1986.

Sutherland SK: Australian animal toxins. Melbourne, 1983, Oxford University Press.

Walker DG: Survival after severe envenomation by the blue-ringed octopus (*Hapalochlaena maculosa*). Med J Aust 2:663-665, 1983.

INDEX